THE HEALTHY MILKSHAKE RECIPES

Fuel Your Body with Nutrient-Dense Beverages

EMMANUEL AKINNODI

TABLE OF CONTENTS

INTRODUCTION

40 DELECTABLE AND DELICIOUS MILKSHAKE RECIPES

12. Raspberry Almond Dream
13. Orange Creamsicle
14. Coffee Lover's Shake
15. Peanut Butter Chocolate Swirl
16. Minty Fresh Shake
17. Strawberry Kiwi Fusion
18. Chocolate Coconut Indulgence
19. Apple Pie Shake
20. Vanilla Date Delight
21. Pina Colada Shake
22. Mixed Nut Power Shake
23. Caramel Apple Drizzle
24. Ginger Turmeric Infusion
25. Mint Chocolate Chip Shake
26. Cherry Almond Bliss
27. Honeydew Melon Refresher
28. Spiced Pumpkin Shake
29. Raspberry Lemon Zest

30. Matcha Green Tea Elixir

31. Blackberry Basil Twist

32. Mocha Banana Fusion

33. Cranberry Orange Delight

34. Maple Walnut Shake

35. Carrot Cake Smoothie

36. Coconut Mango Tango

37. Cucumber Mint Cooler

38. Chocolate Cherry Bomb

39. Pomegranate Berry Burst

40. Strawberry Rhubarb Medley

CONCLUSION

INTRODUCTION

In a world where fad diets come and go, it's refreshing to stumble upon an approach that not only promises transformative results but also embraces the joy of indulgence. Welcome to the tantalizing world of "The Healthy Milkshake Recipes." This groundbreaking book invites you to reimagine your perception of dieting, showing you how deliciousness and nutritional excellence can effortlessly coexist within the confines of a milkshake.

Gone are the days of bland and uninspiring diet regimes that leave you feeling deprived and discouraged. Instead, "The Healthy Milkshake Recipes" beckons you into a realm where wholesome ingredients and mouthwatering flavors meld to create a symphony of taste that leaves you not only satisfied but energized. This book serves as your ultimate guide to achieving your health and wellness goals while savoring every velvety sip.

Harnessing the wisdom of nutrition science and the art of gastronomy, "The Healthy Milkshake Recipes" navigates you through a journey of nourishment that transcends conventional boundaries. Within these pages, you'll discover an array of meticulously crafted milkshake recipes that are as diverse as they are delectable. From antioxidant-rich berry blends to protein-packed nut butter concoctions, each recipe is a testament to the notion that vibrant health doesn't require sacrificing taste.

Moreover, this book isn't just about the ingredients—it's about a mindset shift. The Healthy Milkshake Recipes" empowers you to embrace a more balanced relationship with food. No longer will you view milkshakes as guilty pleasures, but as intentional choices that align with your wellness aspirations.

Whether you're embarking on a weight loss journey, seeking to boost your energy levels, or simply eager to explore a tastier avenue towards wellness, "The Healthy Milkshake Recipes" beckons you with open arms. This isn't just a diet; it's a transformative lifestyle that invites you to sip your way to a healthier, more vibrant you. So, turn the page, fire up your blender, and prepare to embark on a flavorful adventure that promises to redefine how you perceive both milkshakes and the path to optimal health.

40 DELECTABLE AND DELICIOUS MILKSHAKE RECIPES

1. Classic Strawberry Bliss

Ingredients:

1 cup strawberries

1 banana

1 cup almond milk

1 scoop protein powder, ice.

Preparation:

Blend all ingredients until smooth.

Add ice for desired consistency.

2. Chocolate Peanut Butter Delight

Ingredients:

1 tbsp cocoa powder

2 tbsp peanut butter

1 banana

1 cup skim milk, ice.

Preparation:

Blend cocoa, peanut butter, banana, and milk until creamy.

Add ice and blend again.

3. *Green Power Shake*

Ingredients:

1 cup spinach

1/2 cucumber

1/2 avocado

1/2 lemon

1 cup water, ice

Preparation:

Blend spinach, cucumber, avocado, lemon, and water until smooth.

Add ice and blend.

4. Blueberry Blast

Ingredients:

1 cup blueberries

1/2 cup Greek yogurt

1/2 cup almond milk

1 tbsp honey, ice

Preparation:

Blend blueberries, yogurt, almond milk, and honey.

Add ice and blend until creamy.

5. Mango Tango

Ingredients:

1 ripe mango

1/2 cup coconut milk

1/2 cup water

1 scoop vanilla protein powder, ice

Preparation:

Blend mango, coconut milk, water, and protein powder.

Add ice and blend until smooth.

6. Banana Nut Shake

Ingredients:

1 banana

2 tbsp walnuts

1 cup milk (of choice)

1 tsp honey, ice

Preparation:

Blend banana, walnuts, milk, and honey.

Add ice and blend until creamy.

7. Tropical Paradise

Ingredients:

1/2 cup pineapple chunks

1/2 banana

1/4 cup Greek yogurt

1/4 cup coconut water, ice

Preparation:

Blend pineapple, banana, yogurt, and coconut water.

Add ice and blend.

8. Cinnamon Roll Shake

Ingredients:

1/2 tsp cinnamon

1/2 cup oats

1 banana

1 cup milk (of choice)

1 tbsp almond butter, ice

Preparation:

Blend cinnamon, oats, banana, milk, and almond butter.

Add ice and blend until smooth.

9. Vanilla Berry Swirl

Ingredients:

1 cup mixed berries

1/2 tsp vanilla extract

1/2 cup cottage cheese

1 cup almond milk, ice

Preparation:

Blend berries, vanilla extract, cottage cheese, and almond milk.

Add ice and blend.

10. Peachy Keen Shake

Ingredients:

1 ripe peach

1/2 cup plain yogurt

1/2 cup water

1 scoop protein powder, ice

Preparation:

Blend peach, yogurt, water, and protein powder.

Add ice and blend until creamy.

11. Chai Spice Infusion

Ingredients:

1 chai tea bag (brewed and cooled)

1/2 banana

1/4 cup oats

1 cup milk (of choice), ice

Preparation:

Blend cooled chai tea, banana, oats, and milk.

Add ice and blend.

12. Raspberry Almond Dream

Ingredients:

1 cup raspberries

2 tbsp almond butter

1 cup coconut milk

1 tsp honey, ice

Preparation:

Blend raspberries, almond butter, coconut milk, and honey.

Add ice and blend until smooth.

13. Orange Creamsicle

Ingredients:

1 orange (peeled and segmented)

1/2 cup Greek yogurt

1/2 cup milk (of choice), ice

Preparation:

Blend orange segments, yogurt, and milk.

Add ice and blend until creamy.

14. Coffee Lover's Shake

Ingredients:

1/2 cup cold brewed coffee

1/2 banana

1 scoop chocolate protein powder

1 cup almond milk, ice

Preparation:

Blend coffee, banana, protein powder, and almond milk.

Add ice and blend.

15. Peanut Butter Chocolate Swirl

Ingredients:

1 tbsp cocoa powder

2 tbsp peanut butter

1 banana

1/2 cup cottage cheese

1 cup milk (of choice), ice

Preparation:

Blend cocoa, peanut butter, banana, cottage cheese, and milk.

Add ice and blend until smooth.

16. *Minty Fresh Shake*

Ingredients:

1/4 cup fresh mint leaves

1/2 cup spinach

1/2 banana

1/2 cup water

1 scoop protein powder, ice

Preparation:

Blend mint leaves, spinach, banana, water, and protein powder.

Add ice and blend.

17. Strawberry Kiwi Fusion

Ingredients:

1 cup strawberries

1 kiwi (peeled and sliced)

1/2 cup Greek yogurt

1/2 cup water, ice

Preparation:

Blend strawberries, kiwi, yogurt, and water.

Add ice and blend until creamy.

18. Chocolate Coconut Indulgence

Ingredients:

1 tbsp cocoa powder

2 tbsp shredded coconut

1/2 banana

1 cup coconut milk, ice

Preparation:

Blend cocoa, shredded coconut, banana, and coconut milk.

Add ice and blend until smooth.

19. *Apple Pie Shake*

Ingredients:

1 apple (cored and sliced)

1/4 tsp cinnamon

1/4 tsp nutmeg

1/2 cup Greek yogurt

1 cup milk (of choice), ice

Preparation:

Blend apple slices, cinnamon, nutmeg, yogurt, and milk.

Add ice and blend.

20. Vanilla Date Delight

Ingredients:

2 dates (pitted)

1/2 tsp vanilla extract

1/2 cup cottage cheese

1 cup milk (of choice), ice

Preparation:

Blend dates, vanilla extract, cottage cheese, and milk.

Add ice and blend until creamy.

21. Pina Colada Shake

Ingredients:

1/2 cup pineapple chunks

1/4 cup coconut cream

1/2 banana

1/2 cup water, ice

Preparation:

Blend pineapple, coconut cream, banana, and water.

Add ice and blend.

22. Mixed Nut Power Shake

Ingredients:

1 tbsp mixed nuts (almonds, cashews, walnuts)

1 banana

1 cup milk (of choice)

1 scoop protein powder, ice

Preparation:

Blend mixed nuts, banana, milk, and protein powder.

Add ice and blend until smooth.

23. Caramel Apple Drizzle

Ingredients:

1 apple (cored and sliced)

1 tbsp caramel sauce

1/2 cup Greek yogurt

1/2 cup milk (of choice), ice

Preparation:

Blend apple slices, caramel sauce, yogurt, and milk.

Add ice and blend until creamy.

24. Ginger Turmeric Infusion

Ingredients:

1/2 inch ginger root (peeled)

1/2 tsp turmeric powder

1/2 banana

1 cup coconut milk, ice

Preparation:

Blend ginger root, turmeric powder, banana, and coconut milk.

Add ice and blend until smooth.

25. Mint Chocolate Chip Shake

Ingredients:

1/4 cup fresh mint leaves

1 tbsp cocoa nibs

1/2 banana

1/2 cup Greek yogurt

1 cup almond milk, ice

Preparation:

Blend mint leaves, cocoa nibs, banana, yogurt, and almond milk.

Add ice and blend.

26. Cherry Almond Bliss

Ingredients:

1/2 cup cherries (pitted)

2 tbsp almond butter

1/2 cup Greek yogurt

1 cup almond milk, ice

Preparation:

Blend cherries, almond butter, yogurt, and almond milk.

Add ice and blend until creamy.

27. Honeydew Melon Refresher

Ingredients:

1 cup honeydew melon chunks

1/2 cup coconut water

1/2 banana

1 scoop vanilla protein powder, ice

Preparation:

Blend honeydew melon, coconut water, banana, and protein powder.

Add ice and blend.

28. Spiced Pumpkin Shake

Ingredients:

1/2 cup pumpkin puree

1/2 tsp pumpkin spice

1/2 banana

1 cup milk (of choice), ice

Preparation:

Blend pumpkin puree, pumpkin spice, banana, and milk.

Add ice and blend until smooth.

29. Raspberry Lemon Zest

Ingredients:

1 cup raspberries,

Zest of 1 lemon

1/2 cup plain yogurt

1/2 cup water, ice

Preparation:

Blend raspberries, lemon zest, yogurt, and water.

Add ice and blend until creamy.

30. Matcha Green Tea Elixir

Ingredients:

1 tsp matcha green tea powder

1/2 banana

1/2 cup coconut milk

1/2 cup water, ice

Preparation:

Blend matcha powder, banana, coconut milk, and water.

Add ice and blend until smooth.

31. Blackberry Basil Twist

Ingredients:

1 cup blackberries

1/4 cup fresh basil leaves

1/2 cup plain yogurt

1/2 cup water, ice

Preparation:

Blend blackberries, basil leaves, yogurt, and water.

Add ice and blend until creamy.

32. Mocha Banana Fusion

Ingredients:

1/2 ripe banana

1 tbsp cocoa powder

1 shot of espresso (cooled)

1/2 cup milk (of choice), ice

Preparation:

Blend banana, cocoa powder, espresso, and milk.

Add ice and blend.

33. Cranberry Orange Delight

Ingredients:

1/2 cup cranberries

Zest of 1 orange

1/2 banana

1/2 cup Greek yogurt

1/2 cup water, ice

Preparation:

Blend cranberries, orange zest, banana, yogurt, and water.

Add ice and blend until smooth.

34. Maple Walnut Shake

Ingredients:

1/4 cup walnuts

1 tbsp maple syrup, 1/2 banana

1 cup milk (of choice), ice

Preparation:

Blend walnuts, maple syrup, banana, and milk.

Add ice and blend until creamy.

35. Carrot Cake Smoothie

Ingredients:

1/2 cup grated carrot

1/4 tsp cinnamon

1/4 tsp nutmeg

1/2 banana

1 cup milk (of choice), ice

Preparation:

Blend grated carrot, cinnamon, nutmeg, banana, and milk.

Add ice and blend.

36. Coconut Mango Tango

Ingredients:

1/2 cup mango chunks

2 tbsp shredded coconut

1/2 cup coconut milk

1/2 cup water, ice

Preparation:

Blend mango chunks, shredded coconut, coconut milk, and water.

Add ice and blend until smooth.

37. Cucumber Mint Cooler

Ingredients:

1/2 cucumber

1/4 cup fresh mint leaves

1/2 cup coconut water

1/2 cup Greek yogurt, ice

Preparation:

Blend cucumber, mint leaves, coconut water, and yogurt.

Add ice and blend.

38. *Chocolate Cherry Bomb*

Ingredients:

1/2 cup cherries (pitted)

1 tbsp cocoa powder

1/2 banana

1 cup almond milk, ice

Preparation:

Blend cherries, cocoa powder, banana, and almond milk.

Add ice and blend until creamy.

39. Pomegranate Berry Burst

Ingredients:

1/2 cup pomegranate seeds

1/2 cup mixed berries

1/2 cup water

1 scoop protein powder, ice

Preparation:

Blend pomegranate seeds, mixed berries, water, and protein powder.

Add ice and blend.

40. Strawberry Rhubarb Medley

Ingredients:

1/2 cup strawberries

1/4 cup rhubarb

1/2 banana

1/2 cup almond milk, ice

Preparation:

Blend strawberries, rhubarb, banana, and almond milk.

Add ice and blend until smooth.

For all recipes, simply blend the ingredients together until smooth. Adjust the amount of ice and liquid to achieve your desired consistency. Feel free to customize the recipes by adding more or less of certain ingredients based on your taste preferences and dietary needs. Enjoy these delicious milkshake diet recipes as part of a balanced and nutritious meal plan.

NOTE: The sugar content of milkshake recipes can vary depending on the ingredients used. If you are concerned about the sugar content of a milkshake recipe, you can try to reduce the amount of sugar by using less ice cream, less fruit, or sugar-free syrups. You can also add healthy ingredients to the milkshake, such as protein powder, chia seeds, or spinach.

It is also important to note that milkshakes are high in calories, so it is important to enjoy them in moderation. A 16-ounce milkshake can contain about 400 calories, so it is best to share it with a friend or family member.

Here are some tips for making healthier milkshakes:

- Use low-fat or fat-free milk or yogurt.
- Use frozen fruit instead of ice cream.
- Add protein powder or chia seeds for extra nutrients.
- Limit the amount of added sugar.
- Enjoy milkshakes in moderation.

CONCLUSION

CONCLUSION

As you reach the final pages of "The Healthy Milkshake Recipes," we hope you're feeling inspired and empowered on your journey to better health and wellness. Throughout this book, we've taken you on a delicious adventure, demonstrating that nutritious eating doesn't have to be bland or restrictive. The milkshake diet is not just about shedding pounds; it's about embracing a lifestyle that harmoniously blends taste, nutrition, and sustainability.

By now, you've discovered the versatility of milkshake-based meals and their potential to satisfy your cravings while keeping you on track towards your goals. We encourage you to take what you've learned and make it your own, experimenting with ingredients and proportions to suit your individual preferences and dietary needs. The Milkshake Recipes offers you a framework that is both flexible and effective, allowing you to tailor it to your unique journey.

Remember, the journey to a healthier you is not solely defined by the numbers on a scale, but by the choices you make every day. It's about embracing a positive relationship with food, finding joy in the nourishment you provide your body, and celebrating the progress you achieve along the way. As you continue to incorporate these nutritious milkshake recipes into your routine, we invite you to savor the flavors, delight in the variety, and revel in the benefits of a lifestyle that promotes wellness from within.

Your commitment to this journey is commendable, and we believe in your ability to create a sustainable, wholesome lifestyle that reflects the principles of balance, moderation, and self-care. The Milkshake Recipes isn't just a diet – it's a foundation for a life lived to its fullest, where health and pleasure coexist harmoniously.

Thank you for embarking on this transformative path with us. We wish you all the best as you continue to savor each sip and savor each step on your ongoing journey towards health, happiness, and vitality. Here's to a brighter, healthier future – cheers to you!

www.ingramcontent.com/pod-product-compliance
Lightning Source LLC
Chambersburg PA
CBHW080734260726
48660CB00010B/3833